Theo's Story

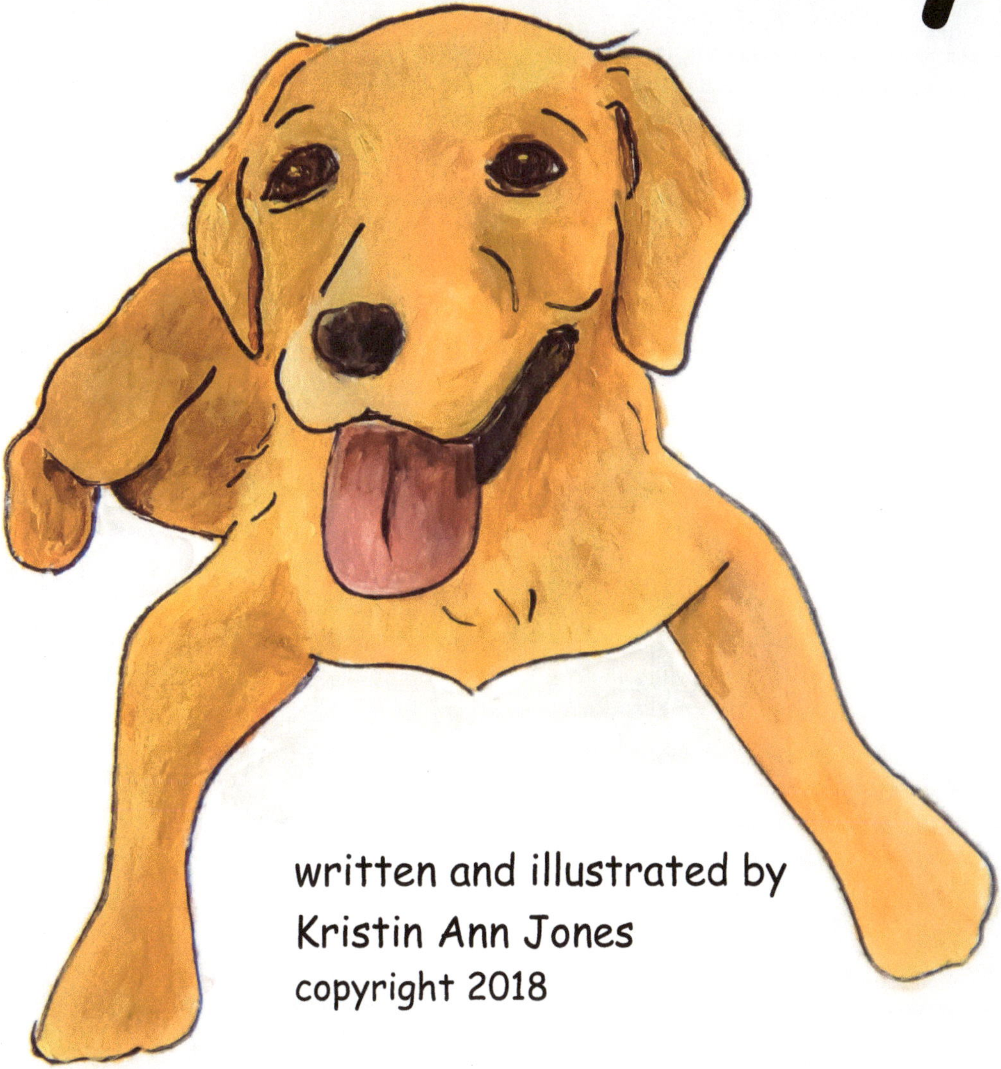

written and illustrated by
Kristin Ann Jones
copyright 2018

This is a story about a dog named Theo and his journey. Theo is a two year old golden retriever who was born with a cleft palate, which means there was a hole in the roof of his mouth. He couldn't eat like his brothers and sisters, and each day was a struggle. Theo was very sick and in pain, but he was brave every day, and finally was able to have surgery to fix the cleft palate. Through the love and support of friends and family, Theo is now a happy, loving, and energetic boy who enjoys the company of everyone. Theo is learning to be part of a Therapy Dog Team so he can visit hospitals and give them love and support.

In a small town, on a big piece of land.

Puppies run everywhere, oh, they are grand.

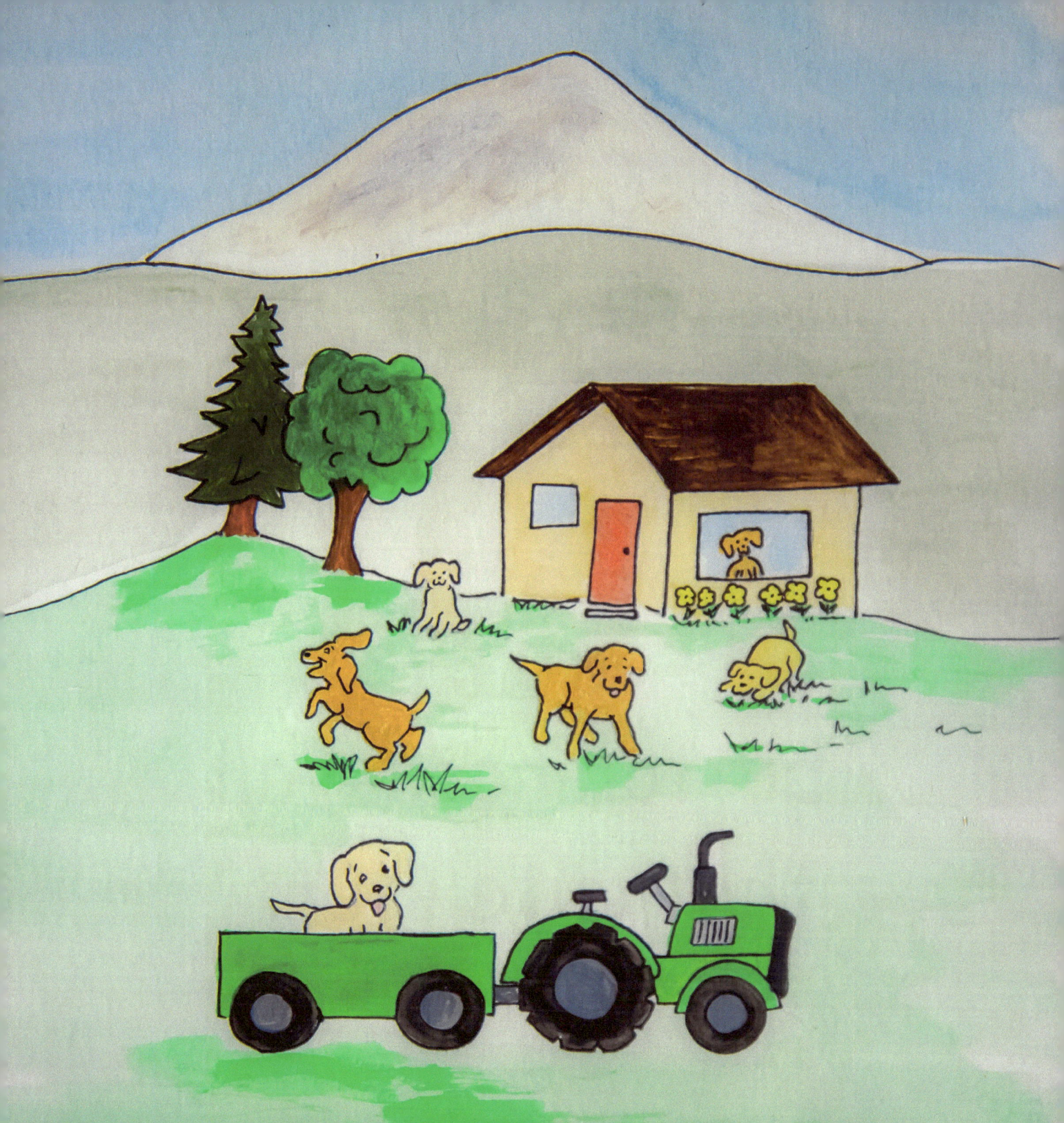

Golden Retrievers, tiny balls of fluff.

Brown eyes, button noses, all that cute stuff.

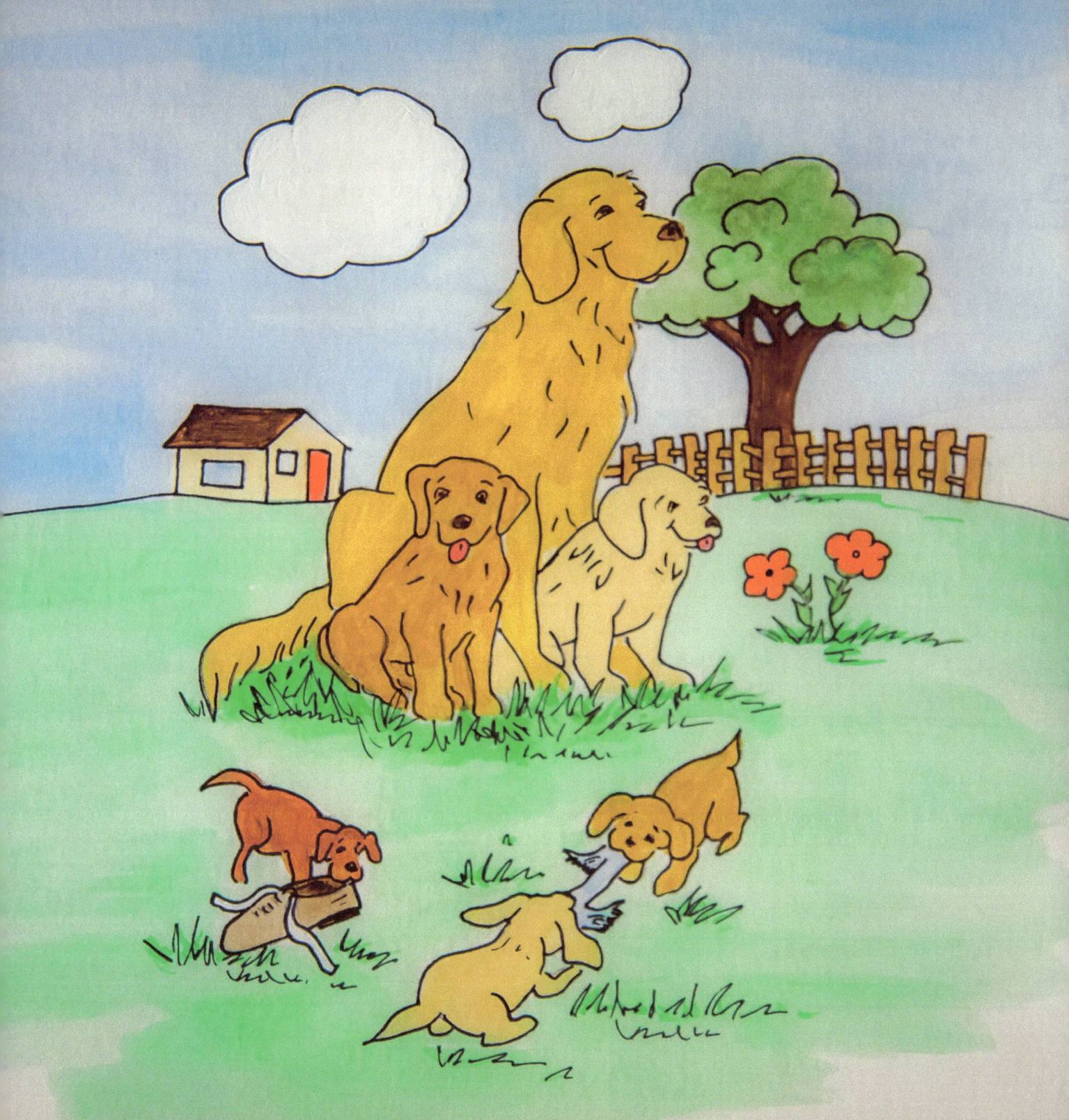

Sometime in June, on a hot summer day.

Puppies were born, and ready to play.

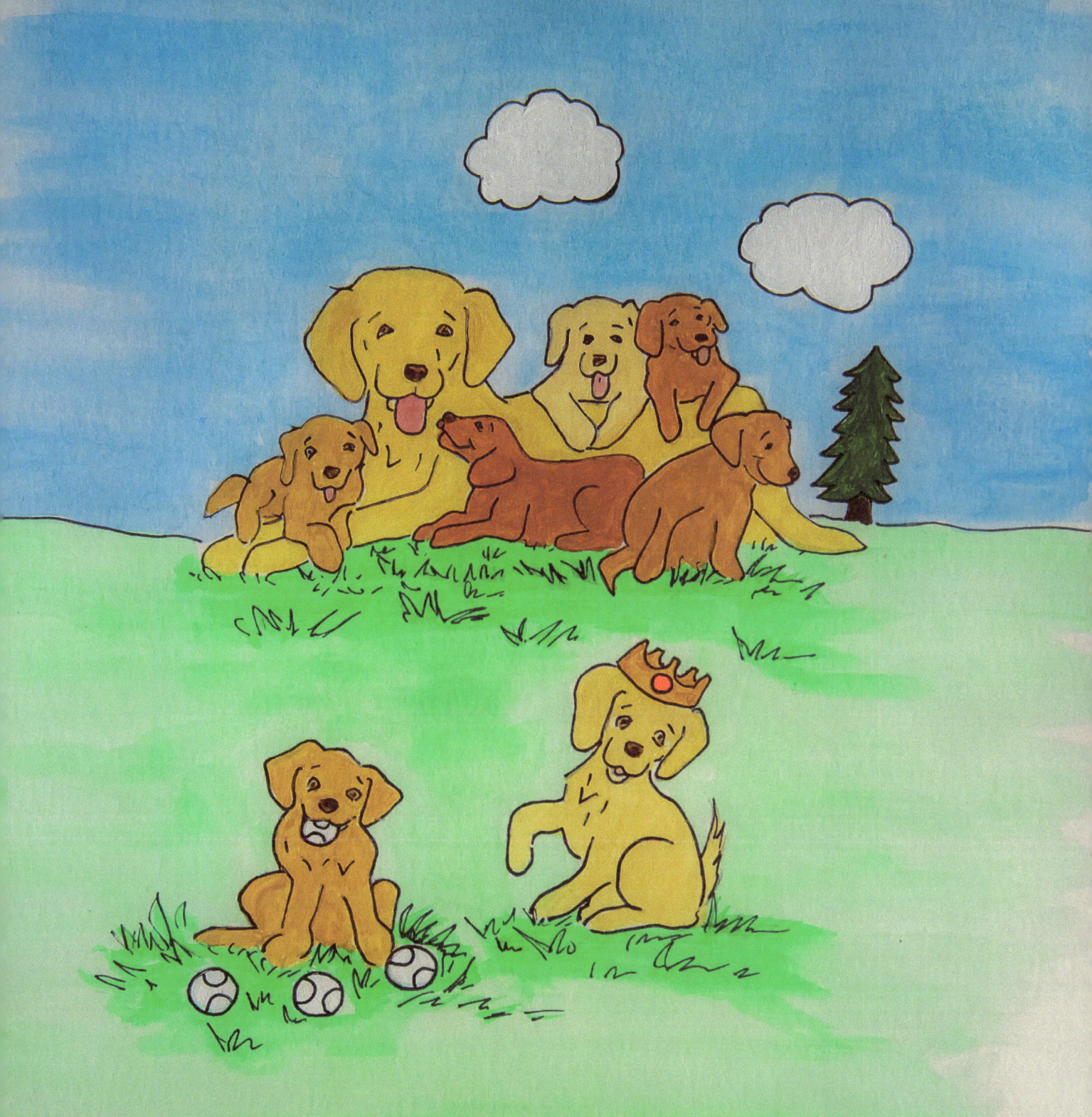

Brothers and sisters, their mom could tell that all were healthy, except one wasn't well.

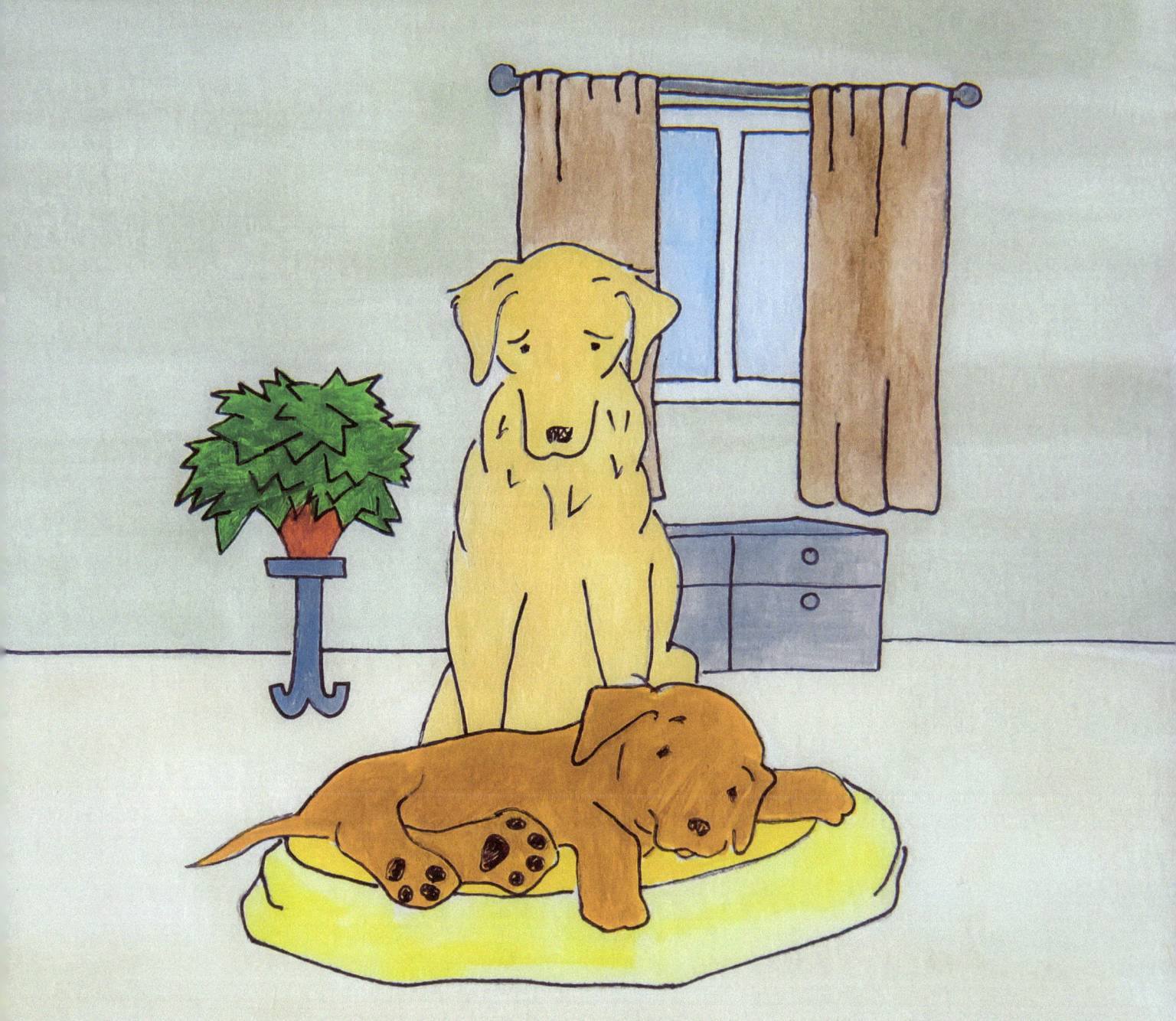

His name was Theo, what a cute boy.

Smiling all the time, and full of sweet joy.

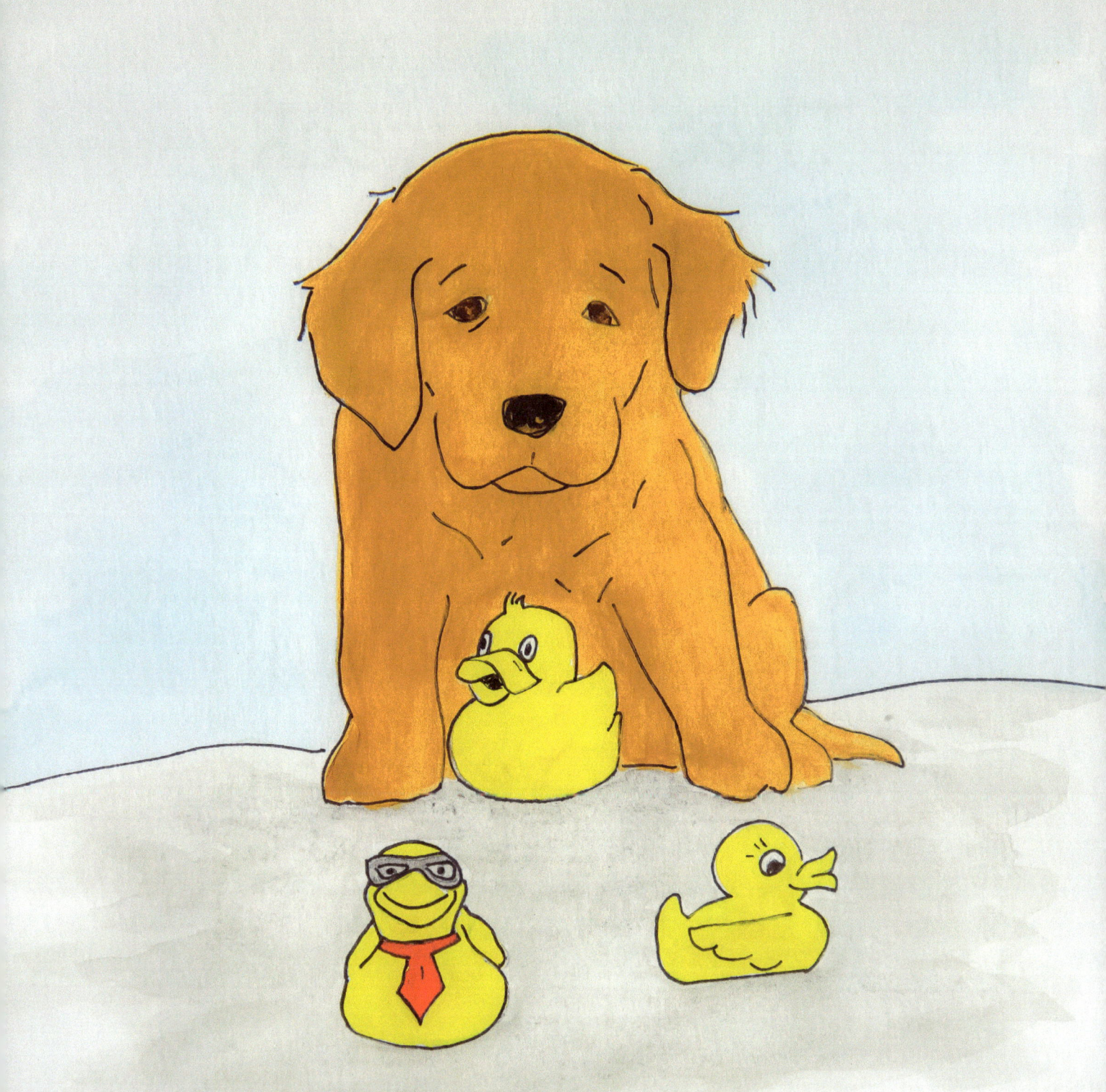

Theo felt weak, despite his huge heart.

He had the will to survive, from the very start.

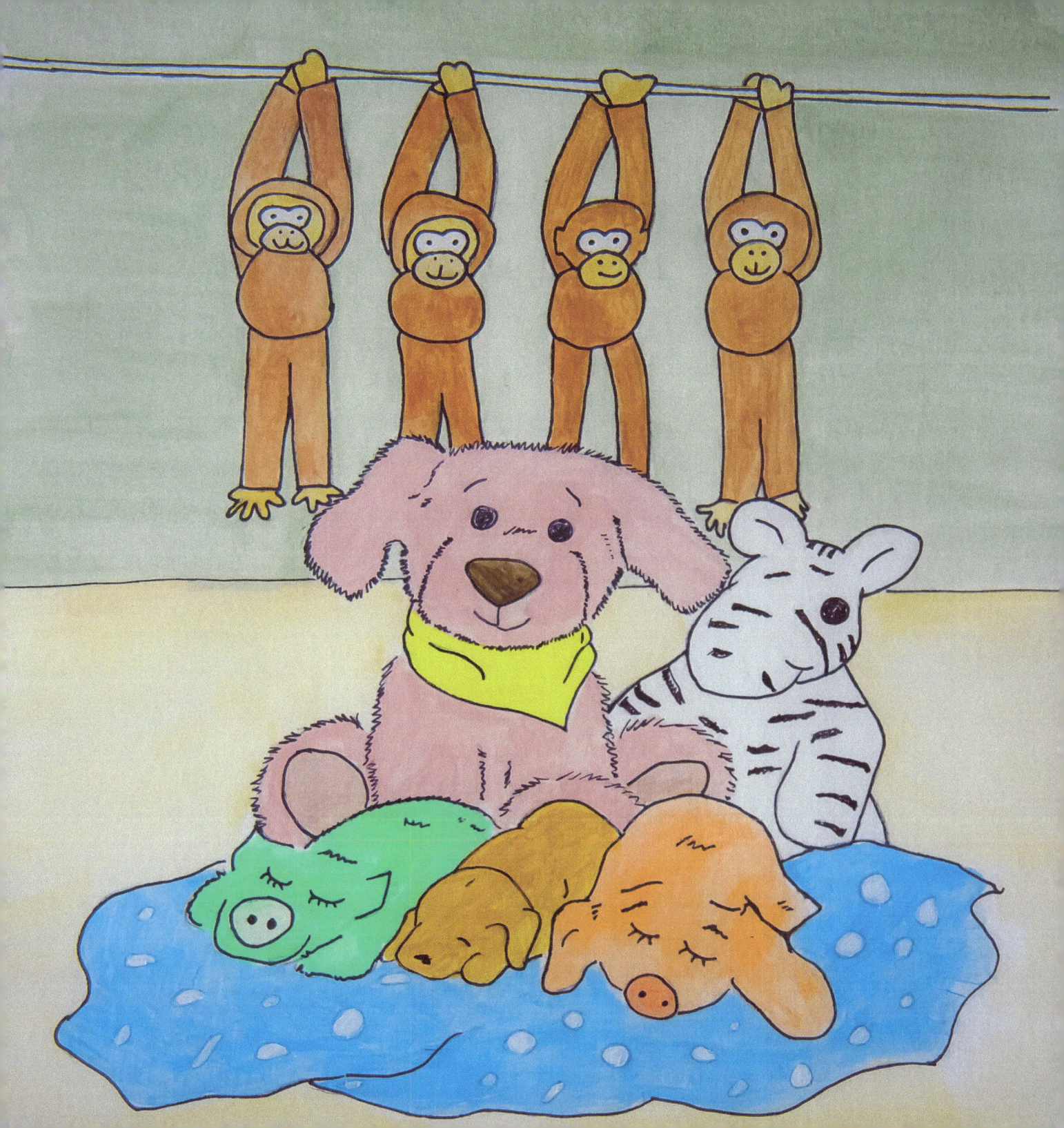

He had a hole in his mouth, the doctors said.

Theo had to be brave, while he was hand fed.

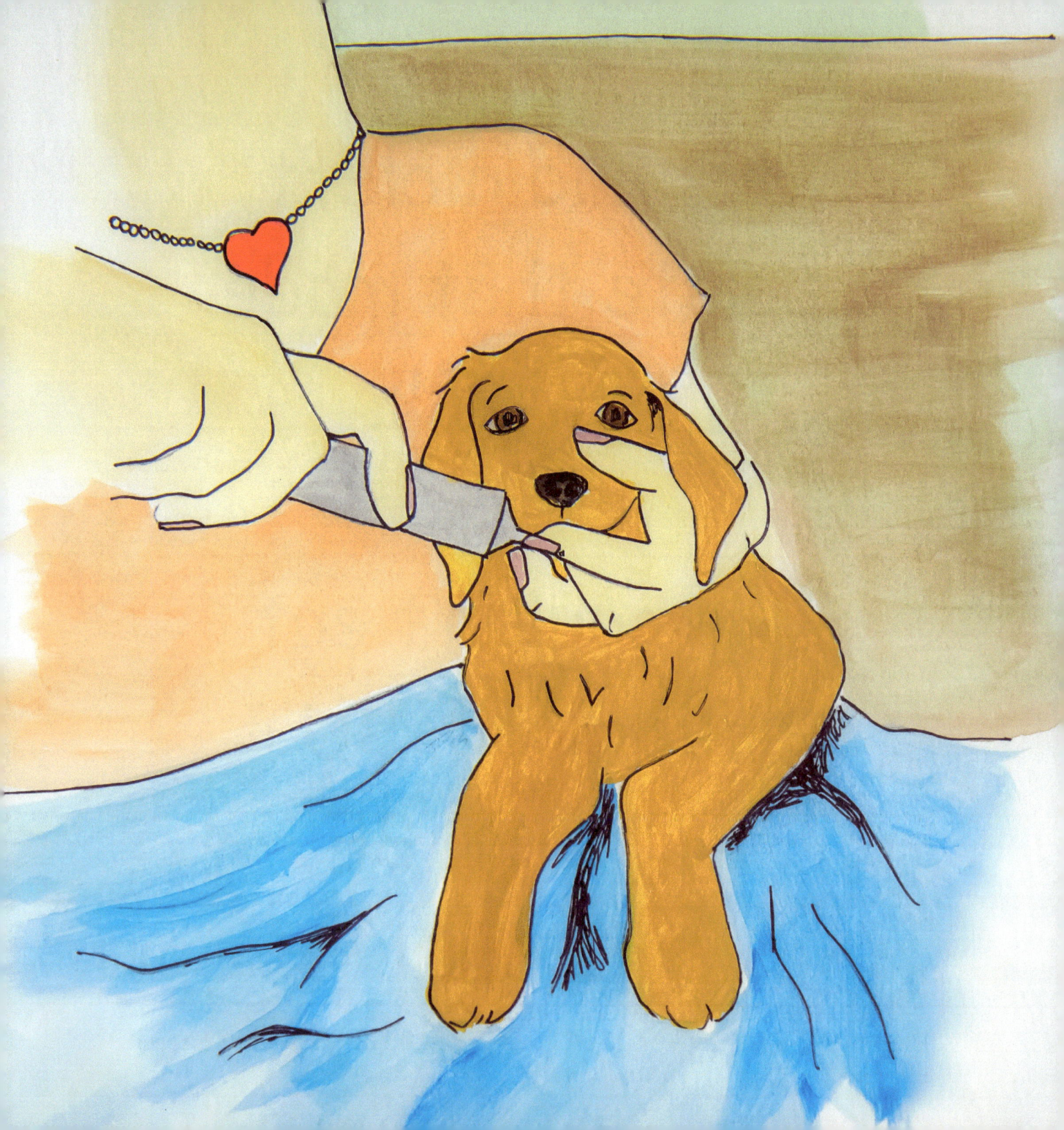

He had a cleft palate that made him sick.

He couldn't eat solid food. BUT IT CAN BE FIXED!

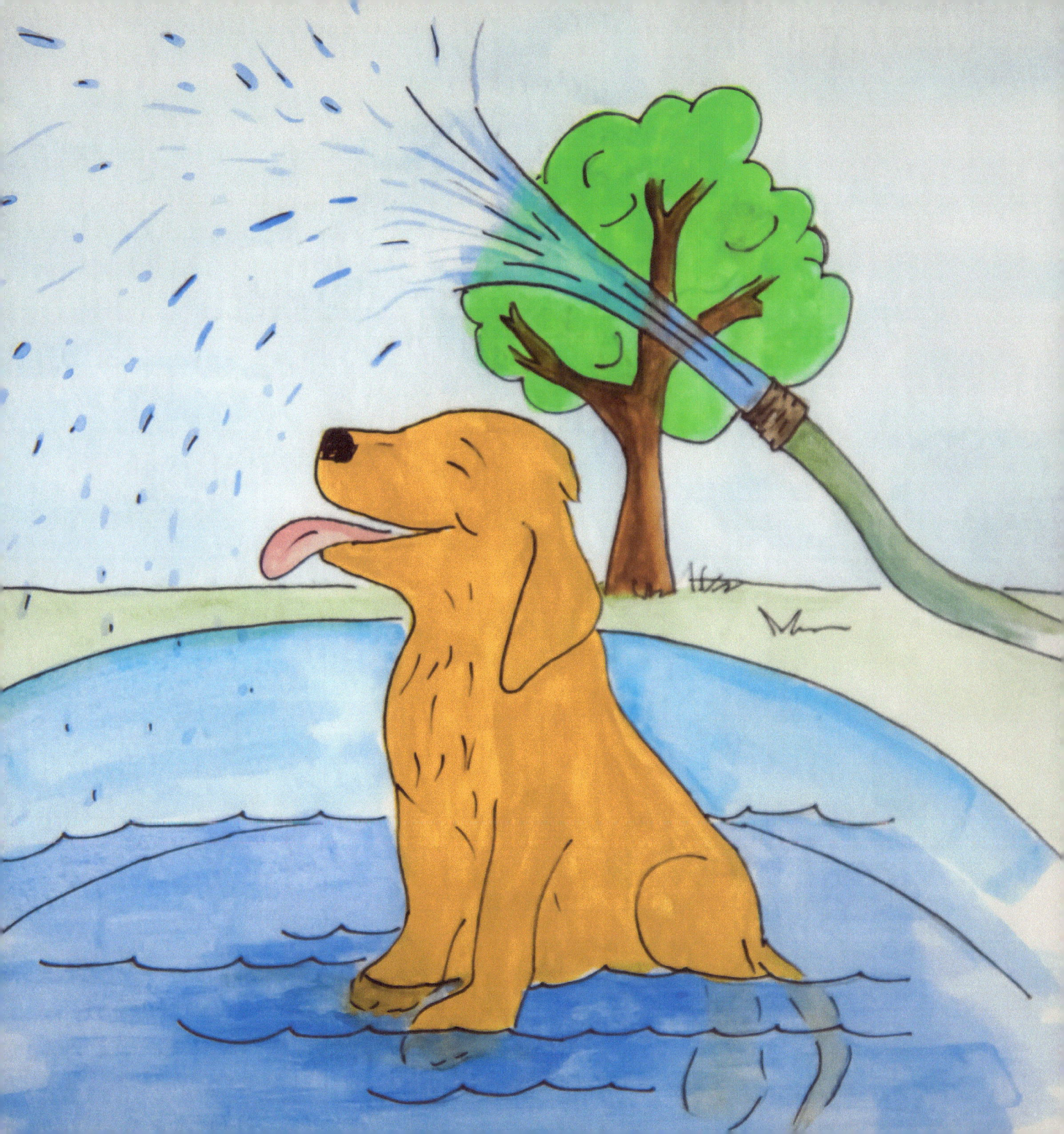

Theo needed surgery to make him all better.

Even though it was scary, it would not last forever.

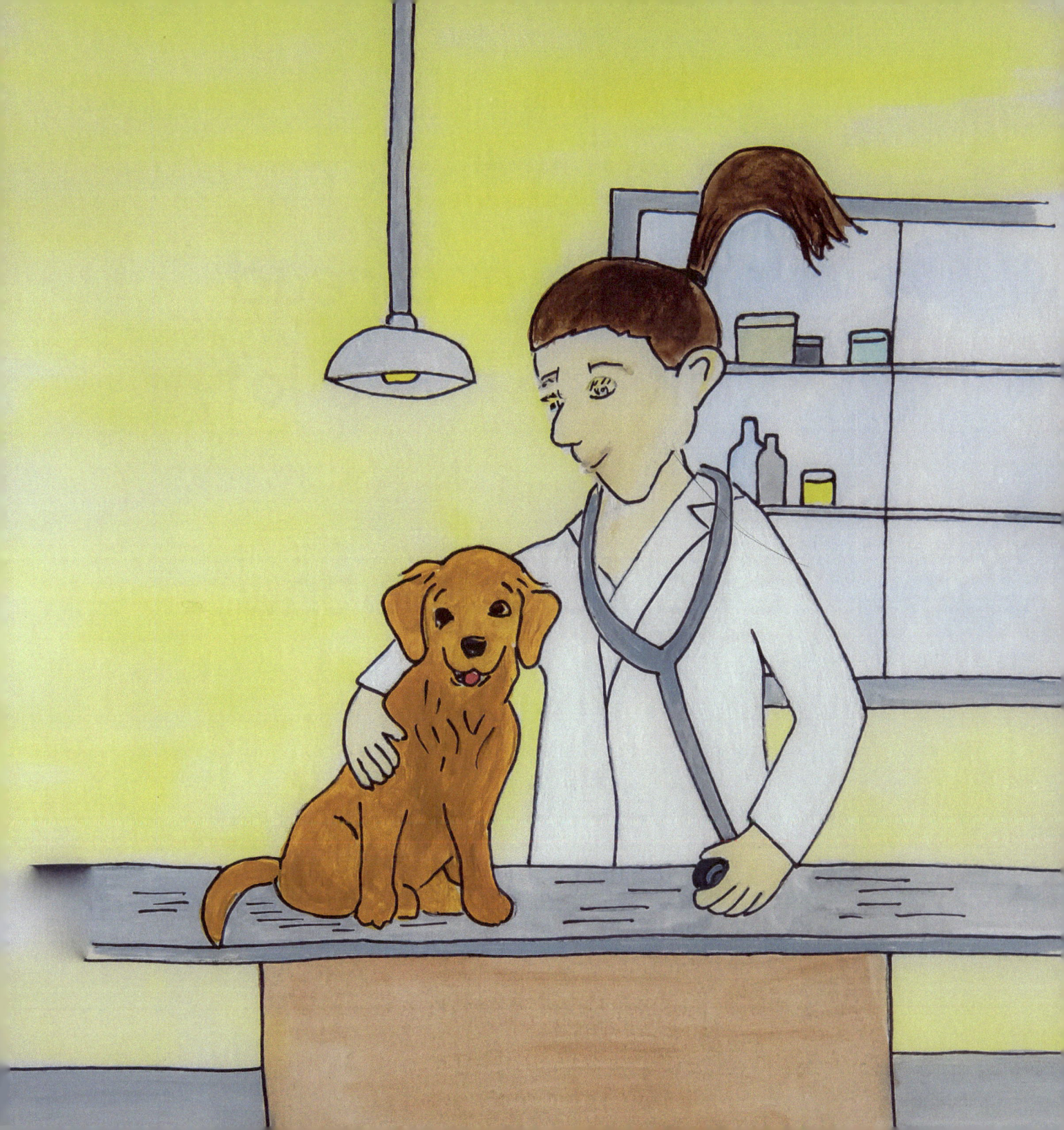

His mom took care of him, and read books to him a lot.

She held his paw, while he got medicine and shots.

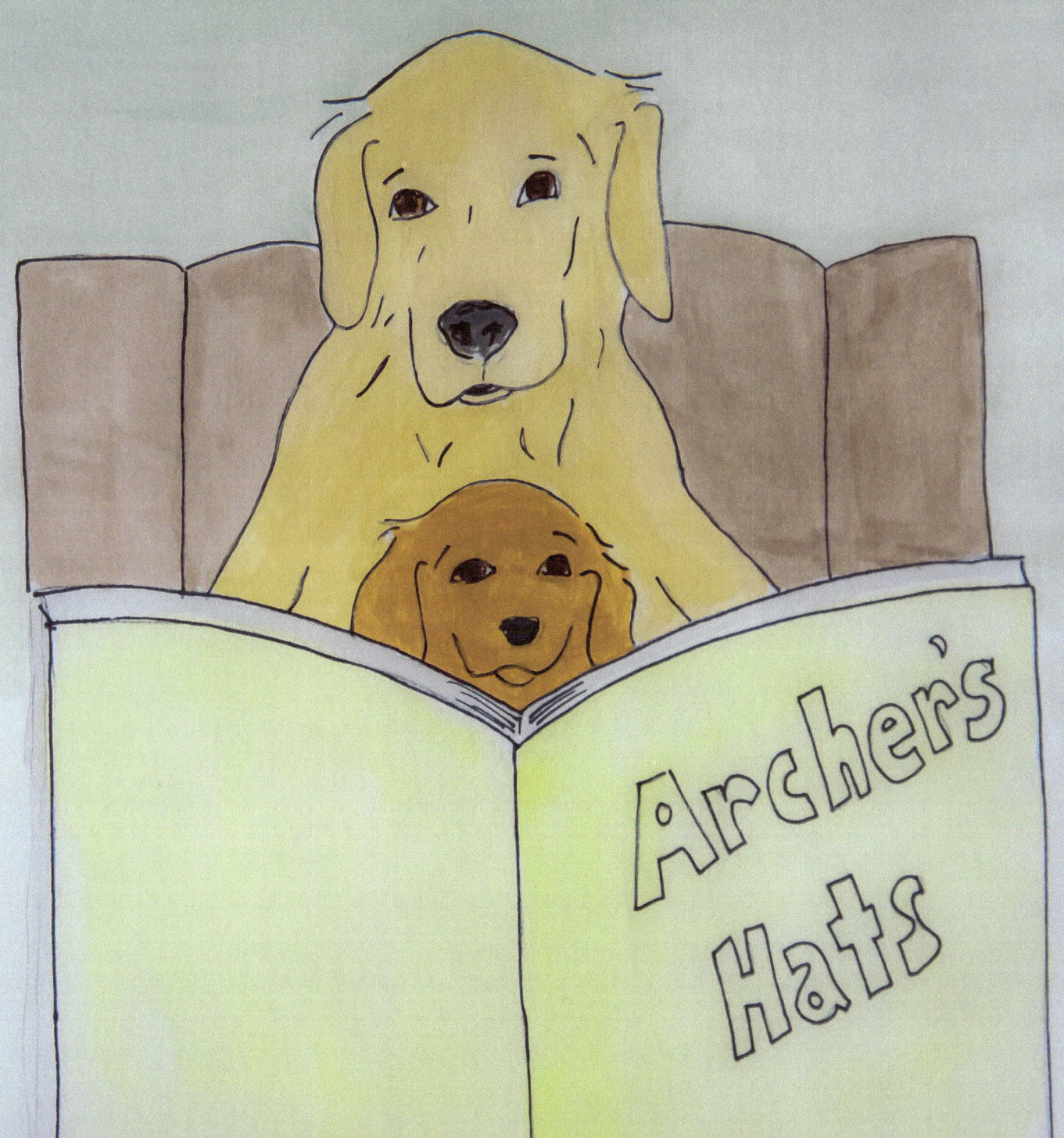

On the day of his surgery, Theo was very strong.

He would be eating food without a tube before too long.

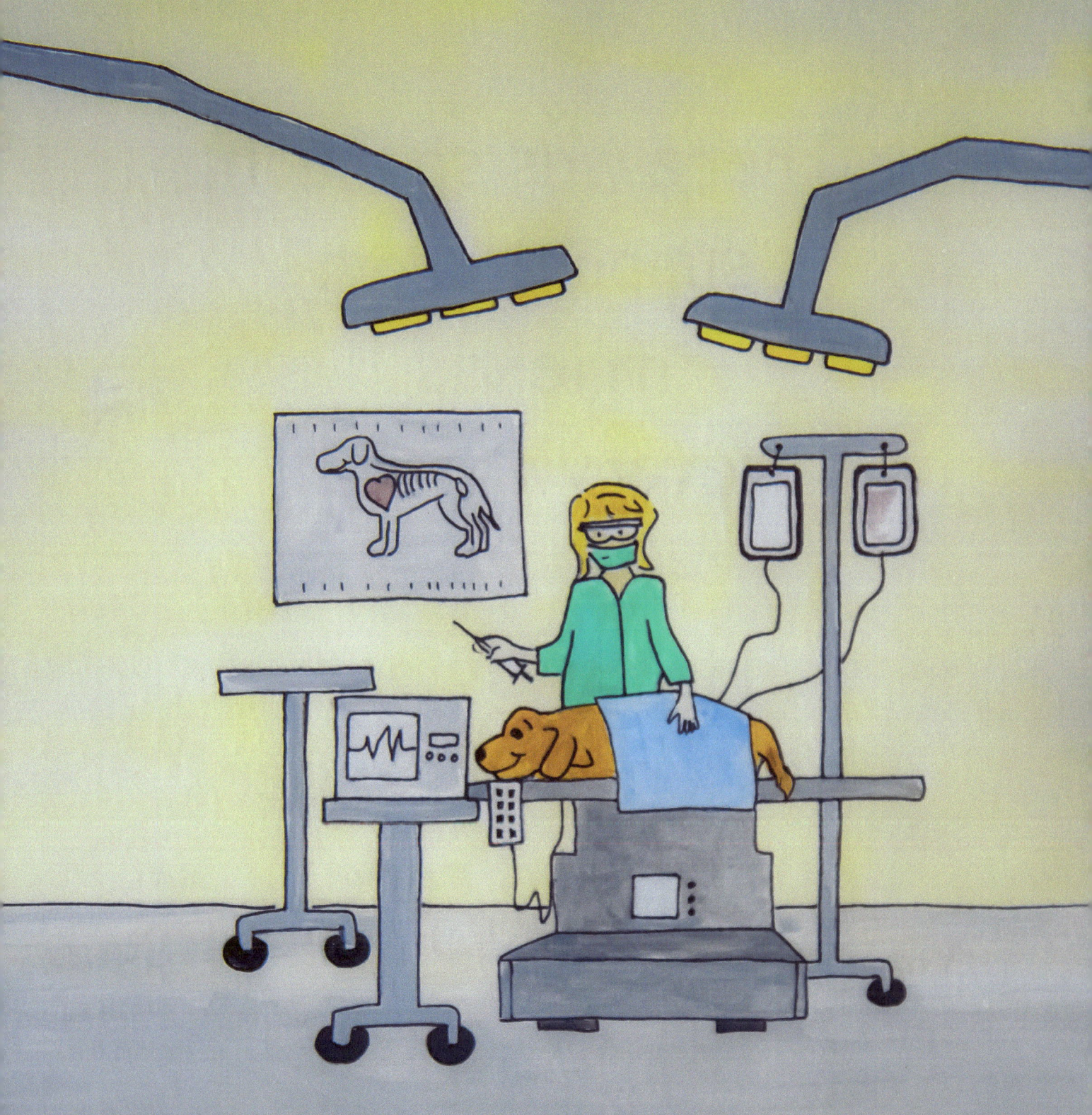

There was so much support from friends everywhere.

He slowly got better with tender love and care.

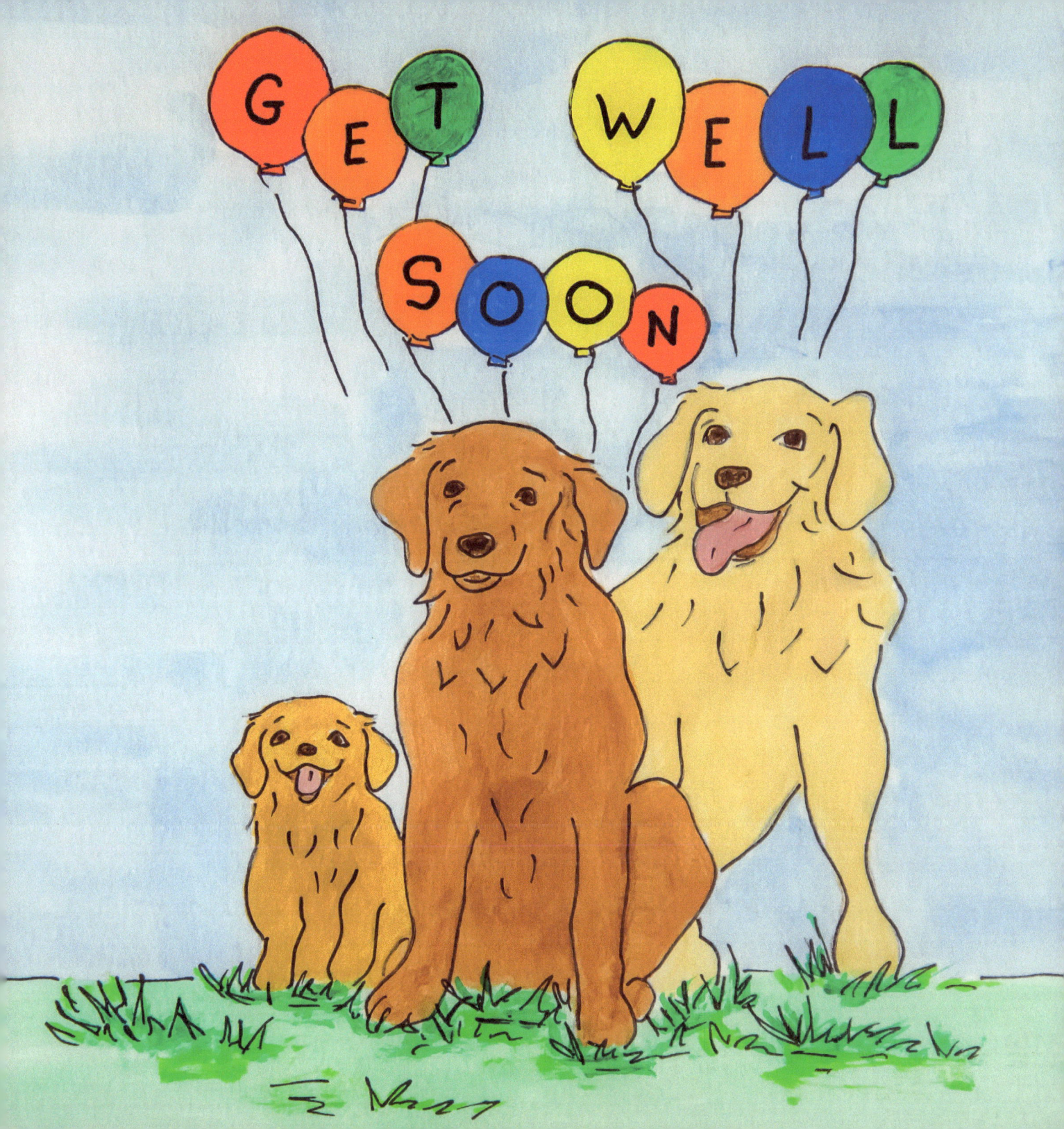

Now Theo can play and run all around.

He has energy to jump high off the ground.

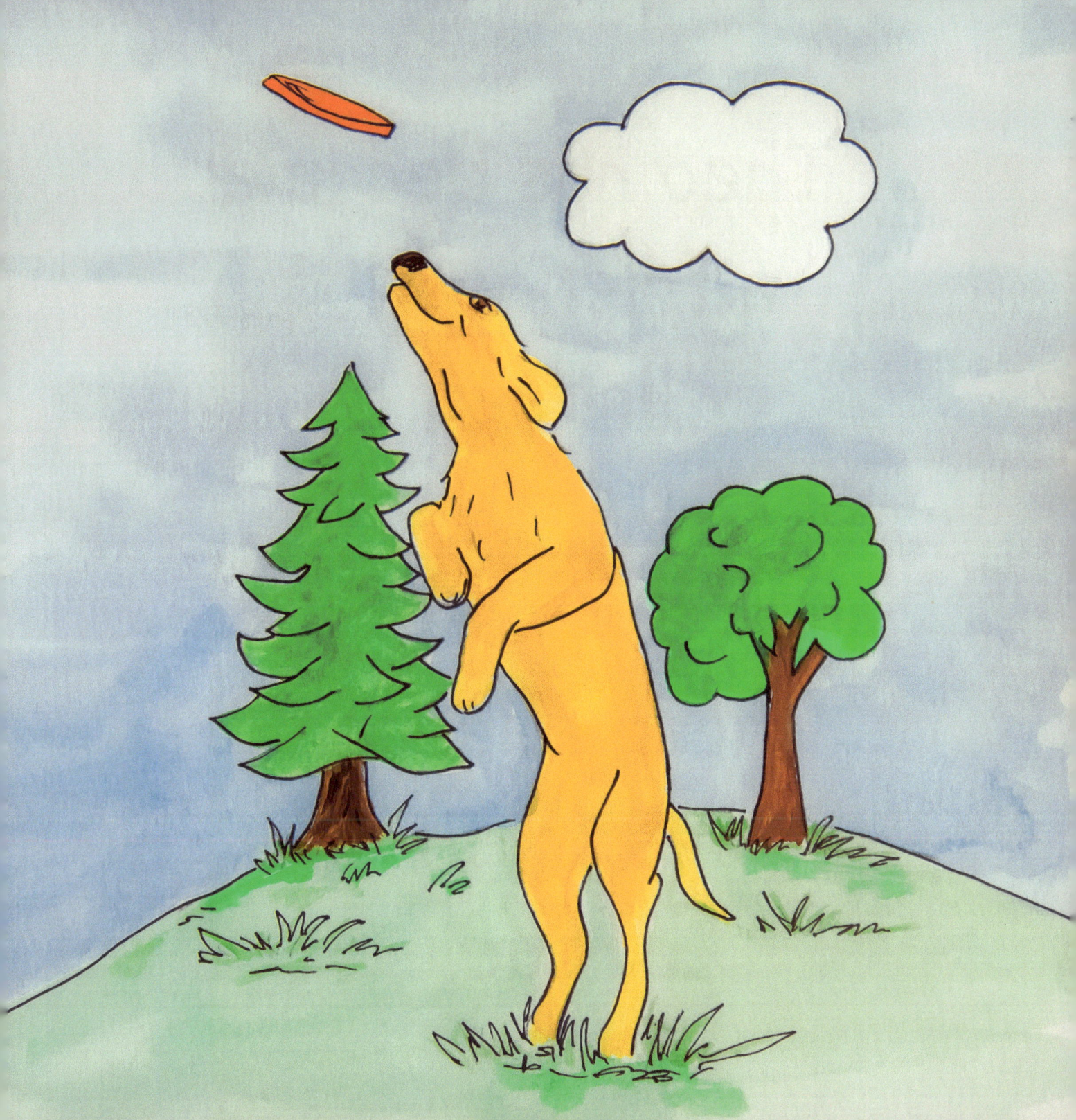

Theo has become a friendly dog indeed.

He visits hospitals, and loves to sit and read.

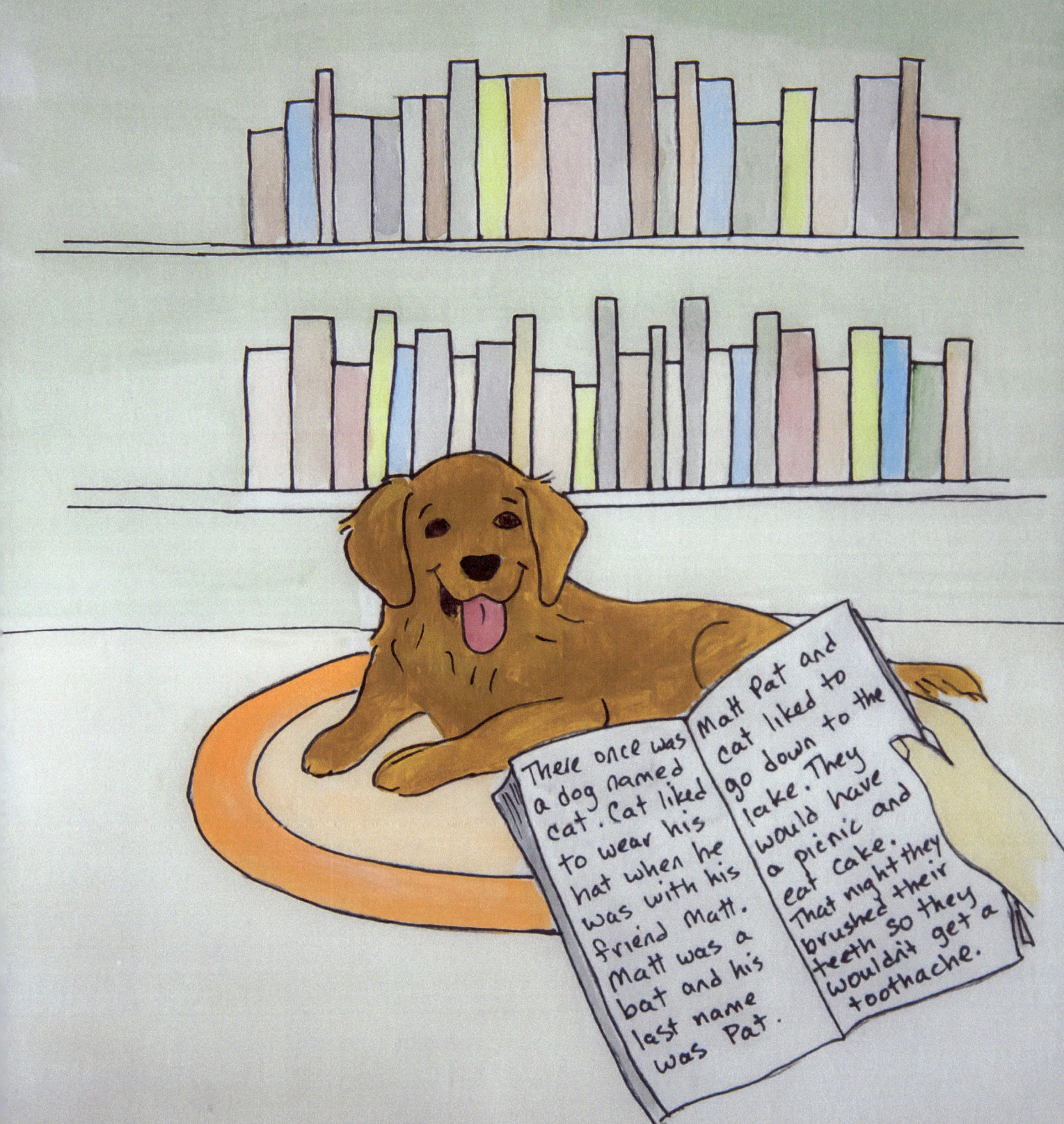

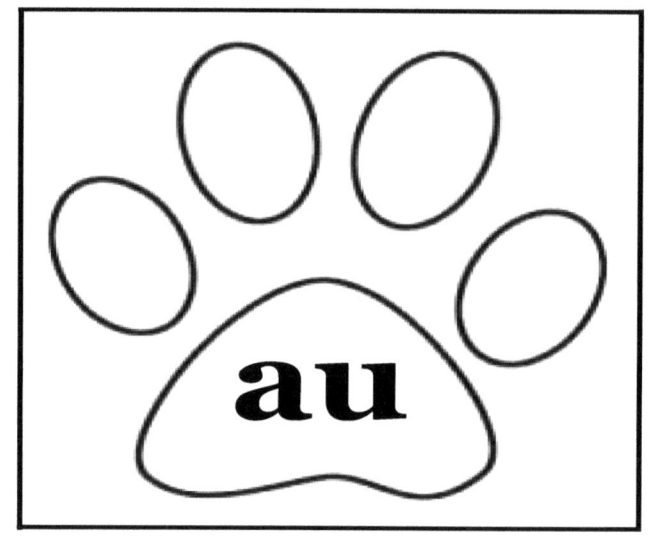

archerunleashed@gmail.com
archerunleashed.com

www.ingramcontent.com/pod-product-compliance
Lightning Source LLC
Chambersburg PA
CBHW041302180526
45172CB00003B/938